2024 Weight Watcher Diet Cookbook for beginners: The

Healthy Meal plan Recipe

Sharon S. Lent

Scan me

Get more Access to more helpful books

TABLE OF CONTENT

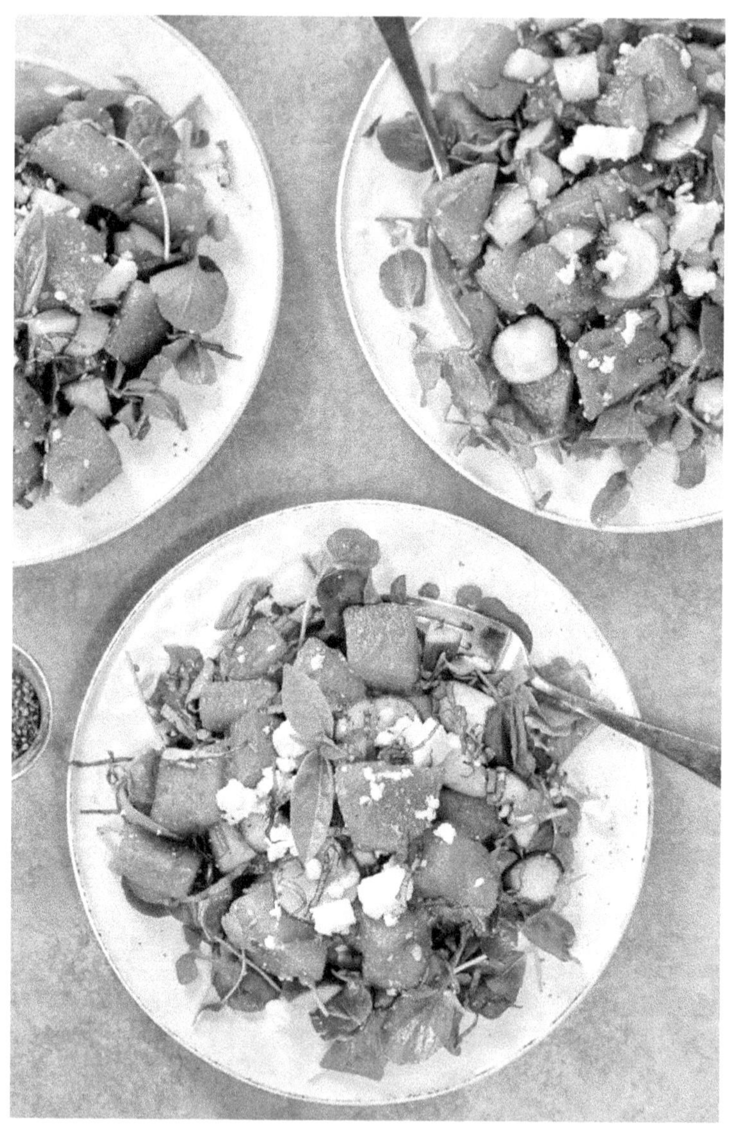

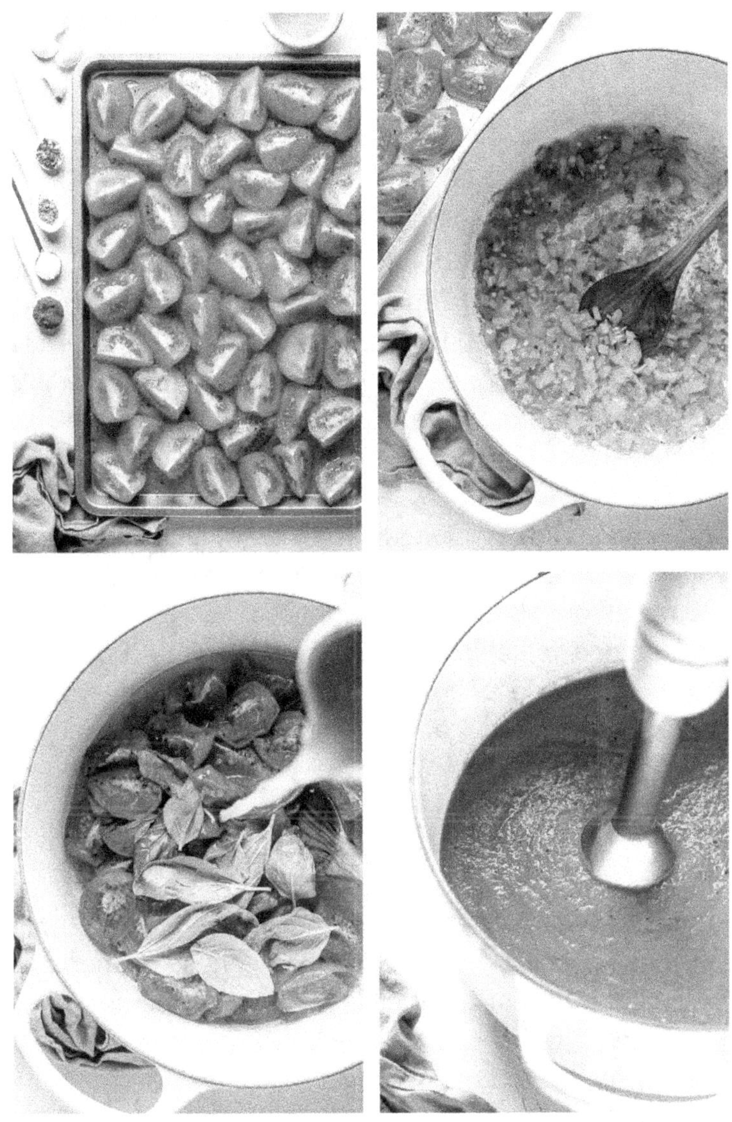

INTRODUCTION
Welcome to weight watcher journey

Dear Fellow Travelers on the Weight Watcher Journey,
As we stand at the threshold of this transformative expedition, let me extend a heartfelt welcome to each one of you. I am Sharon S. Lent, not just your guide but a fellow sojourner on this path to wellness. I invite you to stay put, buckle up, and witness firsthand the incredible metamorphosis that awaits you.

Picture this journey as a captivating adventure, with twists and turns that lead not only to weight loss but to a rediscovery of your true self. I've walked this path, stumbled on some stones, danced through victories, and learned valuable lessons along the way. Allow me to share a glimpse of my own odyssey to inspire you to stay committed and embrace the beautiful transformation that awaits.

Like many of you, I've encountered the ups and downs of battling with excess weight. I've faced the frustration of fad diets and the weariness that comes with unsustainable regimens. It was during those moments of struggle that I realized there had to be a different way a way that embraces individuality, celebrates victories, and makes the journey as important as the destination.

So, here we are, embarking on a journey that transcends the conventional. This is not just about numbers on a scale; it's about reclaiming your vitality, your confidence, and your zest for life. I've been there, questioning if change was possible, and let me assure you, it is. Stay with me, and together we'll uncover the resilience within, transforming challenges into stepping stones toward success.

Let's talk about the power of personalization. I've navigated through the maze of one-size-fits-all approaches and discovered the magic that happens when you tailor your journey to fit your unique needs. It's not just about shedding pounds; it's about crafting a lifestyle that resonates with who you are. Stay committed to the process, and you'll find that the changes you make are not just temporary fixes but lasting upgrades to your well-being.

Community, my fellow travelers, is our secret weapon. I've experienced the incredible support that comes from sharing the journey with like-minded individuals. Together, we form a tribe of encouragement, understanding, and shared victories. Stay connected, share your triumphs and challenges, and witness the power of collective motivation propel you forward.

Now, let's address the celebration of small victories. I've danced in joy over every milestone, whether big or small. These moments aren't just checkpoints; they're the heartbeat of the journey. Embrace each achievement, relish the progress, and you'll find that staying committed becomes a natural part of the adventure.

So, dear friends, as we set forth on this weight watcher journey, I implore you to stay with me. Let's embark on this adventure together, navigating the twists and turns with resilience, celebrating every milestone, and evolving into the best version of ourselves. Welcome to a journey where the destination is just as enchanting as the path we walk. Stay put, and let's watch the magic unfold.

With anticipation and camaraderie,
Sharon S. Lent

CHAPTER 1 : SETTING THE FOUNDATION

As we set out on this tasty odyssey with the Weight Watcher Excursion Cookbook, we should establish the groundwork for a culinary experience that tempts your taste buds as well as makes way for a better, more dynamic way of life. I'm here to direct you through the method involved with creating an establishment that sustains both body and soul.

We should begin with the foundation — fixings. Consider them the structure blocks of your culinary show-stopper. I've strolled the walkways, interpreted marks, and found the specialty of careful shopping for food. Together, we'll investigate the abundance of new produce, lean proteins, and healthy grains that structure the premise of scrumptious, wellbeing cognizant feasts. Prepare to transform your kitchen into a material of dynamic, nutritious potential outcomes.

Presently, we should discuss the craft of arrangement. I've experimented with methods that transform the simplest ingredients into culinary delights as I've danced around kitchens. Go along with me in embracing the delight of cooking — whether you're a carefully prepared culinary expert or a beginner in the kitchen. We will transform your cooking experience into a celebration of creativity and nourishment through simple recipes and cooking advice.

Segment control is our next support point. I've wrestled with the idea, it is vital to grasp that equilibrium. In the Weight Watcher Excursion Cookbook, we'll disentangle the secrets of part estimates, guaranteeing that each plate is an amicable mix of flavors and dietary goodness. There's no need to focus on hardship; it's tied in with enjoying each chomp carefully.

We should not fail to remember the significance of assortment. I've explored through the tedium of redundant feasts and found the delight of variety. The cookbook will be your visa to a universe of tastes, surfaces, and fragrances. Express farewell to culinary fatigue as we investigate a range of dishes that keep your taste buds charmed and your obligation to a better way of life unfaltering.

Dinner arranging is our last foundation. I've encountered the tumult of latest possible moment choices and the quietness of a thoroughly examined plan. Together, we'll create a feast plan that fits consistently into your life, pursuing solid decisions helpful and pleasant. There's really no need to focus on inflexible principles; It involves creating a path to success.

In this way, individual culinary lovers, as we set the establishment for the Weight Watcher Excursion Cookbook, imagine your kitchen as a space where wellbeing and delight merge. I welcome you to go along with me in this gastronomic investigation, where each feast is a stage towards a dynamic, healthy lifestyle. We should make a ton of amazing food, enjoy the excursion, and lay the preparation for a better, more tasty you.

The basic of weight watcher

We should dig into the essentials of the Weight Watchers program an excursion that rises above conventional eating regimens and embraces an all encompassing way to deal with solid living. Go along with me as we disentangle the rudiments, demystifying the quintessence of this extraordinary experience.

Adaptability is a sign of the Weight Watchers reasoning. I've experienced the liberation that comes with flexibility no food is off-limits in contrast to rigid diets. Choosing options that are compatible with your lifestyle and preferences is the key. This flexibility guarantees that your process is feasible and customized to your special requirements.

Past the mathematical perspective, local area support is an indispensable part. I've found comfort and consolation in the Weight Watchers people group, where shared encounters, triumphs, and difficulties make an organization of figuring out people. Embrace this local area, draw motivation, and offer your own victories it's an aggregate excursion toward prosperity.

Mentality matters in the Weight Watchers venture. Moving from a prohibitive mindset to one of self-strengthening and positive decisions is groundbreaking. I've seen the effect of this mentality shift, understanding that it's about the scale as well as developing a sound connection with food and oneself.

Fundamentally, the nuts and bolts of Weight Watchers rotate around careful eating, adaptability, local area support, and a positive outlook. It's not only an eating routine a way of life advances generally prosperity. Join me in embracing these fundamentals and making conscious choices every step of the way toward a happier, healthier you.

Meal planning Strategies

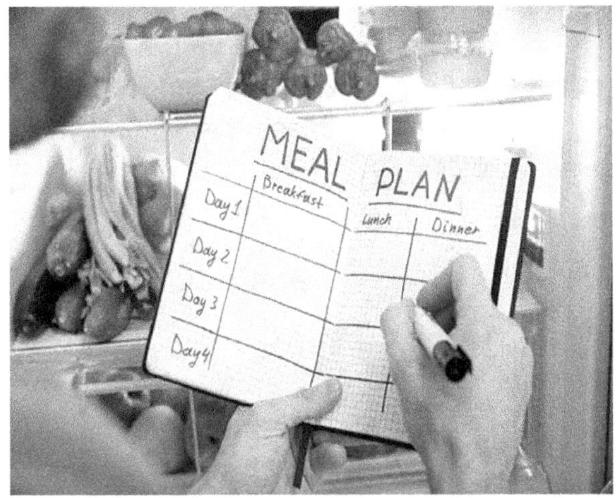

Meal planning is like orchestrating a delicious symphony for your week. Begin by assessing your dietary needs and preferences a personalized overture. Take stock of what's in your **Pantry and fridge :** the opening notes of your composition. Choose recipes that align with your goals, whether it's fitness, weight loss, or simply enjoying diverse cuisines the melody starts to take shape.

Create a shopping list : the instrumental arrangement of ingredients. Allocate time for prep a crucial tempo to maintain. Batch cooking can be your crescendo, saving time and ensuring a harmonious flow throughout the week. Consider the balance of proteins, carbs, and veggies the key to a well-rounded composition.

Flexibility is your adagio; Be open to improvisation and adapt to unforeseen changes. As you savor the final dish, appreciate the masterpiece you've orchestrated – a symphony of flavors, nutrition, and efficiency. Meal planning is your culinary masterpiece, enhancing both your palate and lifestyle.

CHAPTER 2 : BREAKFAST IDEALS

Delicious almond berry smoothie

PREP TIME: 10 mins
Total Time: 10 mins
Servings: 1

INGREDIENTS

1 cup frozen blueberries

1 banana

½ cup almond milk

1 tablespoon almond butter

water as needed

INSTRUCTION

Combine blueberries, banana, almond milk, and almond butter in a blender; blend until smooth, adding water for a thinner smoothie.

SIMPLE ALMOND CEREAL

INGREDIENTS

4 c. rolled oats
1 c. unsweetened large coconut flakes (not shredded)
1 c. whole almonds, roasted and salted
1 c. dried tart cherries
2 tbsp. pure maple syrup, plus more for serving
2 tsp. vanilla extract
1/2 c. pepita seeds, roasted and salted
1 tsp. cinnamon
1 tsp. dried ground ginger
1/2 tsp. allspice
milk, for serving

INSTRUCTIONS

Preheat oven to 350°F.

Spread out the oats evening on a baking sheet, then place the coconut in an even layer over the top. Bake 7 to 11 minutes, watching closely, until the coconut is evenly golden brown. Remove from the oven and allow to cool slightly.

Meanwhile, roughly chop the almonds and cherries.

In a small bowl, combine the maple syrup and vanilla, then heat in the microwave until warmed through and the consistency is thinner, about 20 seconds (alternately, heat on the stovetop).

In a large bowl, combine the toasted oats and coconut with the cherries, almonds, pepitas, cinnamon, ginger, allspice, and the maple-vanilla mixture, and stir to thoroughly combine. Pour the mixture back onto the baking sheet and spread into an even layer to allow the muesli to fully dry, about 10 minutes. Stir to break up any clumps, then transfer to a sealable container.

Serve with milk and a touch of maple syrup.

NOTES
• I like my coconut barely toasted, so I toasted the oats for 7 minutes before adding the coconut on top and toasting 3 minutes more.
• Similarly, I prefer raw nuts and seeds in my breakfast cereal, so I used raw sliced almonds and raw pepita seeds. Then added a pinch of salt to the cereal mixture.
• I added the spices and pinch of salt into the warmed maple syrup and vanilla mixture to evenly coat the oats.
• The spices were warm and delicious. I'm also going to experiment using cinnamon and cardamom next time and maybe a little almond extract. This recipe is versatile like that!
• I added an extra tablespoon of maple syrup (3 tbsp. total) to the cereal to skip adding more before each serving. Call me lazy. It was perfectly sweetened to my tastes, especially with the addition of the dried cherries and coconut.

HOMEMADE CHICKEN OMELET

INGREDIENTS
4 large eggs, beaten
Kosher salt, to taste
Pepper, to taste
1 teaspoon olive oil
1/3 cup shredded cooked chicken
2 tablespoons shredded Gruyere cheese
2 tablespoons chopped spinach
Spinach salad and crusty bread, for serving

INSTRUCTION
Gather your ingredients.

Whisk the eggs until the yolks and whites are completely combined. Add salt and pepper. You can add more to taste later if needed.

Heat the teaspoon of oil in a non-stick or cast-iron skillet on high. Swirl the oil around so that it completely coats the bottom of the pan.

Pour the beaten eggs into the skillet and turn the heat down to low. Swirl the eggs to completely coat the bottom of the pan.

Using a rubber spatula pull the egg from the outside edge into the center, exposing parts of the pan so the egg can cook completely. Then leave the omelette alone for another minute or two. Remember to cook it on low heat so that it does not brown too much.

Warm the chicken slightly in the microwave or on the stovetop before adding it to the omelet—it won't get hot enough to completely heat up all of the chicken.

Add the shredded chicken, shredded gruyere, and chopped spinach to half of the omelet. Cook for 30 seconds.

Fold the other half of the omelet over the top of the filling. Cook for another 30 seconds to a minute, or until the cheese has melted.

Serve with a small spinach salad and some crusty bread.

BREAD ROLL EGG MORNING

INGREDIENTS

slices Bread
5 eggs
Onion & scotch bonnet
Vegetable oil
Seasoning cube, curry & mixed spices
1/4 tsp of salt
Thyme & garlic powder
Flour

INSTRUCTION

Crack the eggs in a clean bowl, add all the spices & chopped onions. In a frying pan, add the grated scotch bonnet & oil to fry, then add up the egg mixture, close for a minute.

Scramble the egg & keep frying until golden brown.

Cut the edges of the bread, roll with a rolling pin, add spread the egg in one side & mat roll it, mix flour with water to achieve a thick batter, use samosa brush to spread the batter at last portion of the bread & mat roll it.

Dip in egg mix with salt & then in cornflakes & dip fry in hot oil, enjoy.

Salmon Green Breakfast

SERVINGS: 2
PREP TIME: 5MINUTES
COOK TIME: 5MINUTES
TOTAL TIME: 10 MINUTES

INGREDIENTS
FOR THE SALMON AND EGGS
4 large eggs
2 tbsp half and half*
1/8 tsp salt
1 tbsp ghee or butter
4 ounces hot roasted smoked salmon** broken into chunks
1/4 cup thinly sliced fresh chives
freshly ground black pepper
COMPATIBLE PAIRINGS
fresh avocado slices
hash browns
drop biscuits

INSTRUCTIONS
In a medium bowl, combine the eggs, half and half, and salt, by using a fork or whisk. Beat until well blended, 30-60 seconds.

Heat a nonstick skillet over medium to medium high heat, and add the ghee or butter.

Add the beaten eggs and use a flat spatula to scrape the bottom of the pan as it cooks, in order to form large curds. This should take 1-2 minutes. When the egg is almost completely cooked, add the chunks of salmon, and keep cooking for another minute, until the egg is cooked and the salmon is warm.

Gently fold in the chives, and grind black pepper on top, to taste. Serve right away, and enjoy!

WATERMELON CHAI SMOOTHIE

Yield: 4
PREP time: 5 MINUTES
Total time: 5 MINUTES

INGREDIENTS
2 cups watermelon
2 cups frozen strawberries
1-2 tablespoons chia seeds
1 tablespoon honey
1 lime (juiced) - about 2 tablespoons
1 tablespoon true lime powder
1 cup ice
½ cup milk (optional)
 1 banana

INSTRUCTIONS
Add all ingredients to blender.
Blend on high until desired smoothie consistency.
Pour into glass for serving and
enjoy!

NOTES
Substitute your strawberries and banana with other fruits
and veggies for endless watermelon fruit combos!

Feel free to substitute fresh lime juice for bottled lime juice if needed. Can also substitute True Lime Powder for lime juice if desired.

If looking for a creamier smoothie we suggest using 2% or whole milk for optimal flavor. But you can use almond or soy milk instead or skip the milk all together!

Add less ice for a thinner consistency. For a thicker smoothie consistency freeze your watermelon beforehand

CINNAMON BANANA SMOOTHIE

Prep Time: 2minutes
Blend time: 2minutes
Total Time: 4minutes
 Servings: 1 serving
Calories: 61 kcal

EQUIPMENT

Blender

INGREDIENTS

2 frozen bananas medium sized
1/2 tsp ground cinnamon
1/2 cup plain greek yogurt
1/2 cup unsweetened vanilla almond milk

INSTRUCTIONS

First, start by cutting and freezing the bananas.
Next, add the frozen bananas, unsweetened vanilla almond milk, plain greek yogurt and ground cinnamon to a blender.
Blend all the ingredients together until smooth.
Finally, top off with more ground cinnamon if desired, serve cold and **enjoy!**

NOTES

If you don't have unsweetened vanilla almond milk, you may use any other kind of milk you have on hand. I've also made this smoothie with oat milk and it was really good!

You can store this smoothie in the refrigerator for up to 2 days in an air tight container. Alternatively, you can make ahead and freeze in an air tight container for up to 3 months.

The sweetness from the bananas was perfect for my taste! However, if you don't think the smoothie is sweet enough, feel free to add a little honey or your sweetener of choice!

CHAPTER 3 : VEGETARIAN AND VEGAN RECIPES

Potato Buttermilk Appetizer

SERVINGS: 6 to 8 servings
PREP TIME: 45 minutes
COOK TIME: 15 minutes
TOTAL TIME: 1 hour

INGREDIENTS

2 cups buttermilk

1 teaspoon hot sauce

2 teaspoons fresh thyme leaves plus more for garnish

3 teaspoons salt divided

2 teaspoon black pepper divided

3 to 4 medium or small Russet potatoes rinsed

2 cups all-purpose flour

2 teaspoons white pepper

1/2 teaspoon basil

1 teaspoon celery salt

1 teaspoon dried mustard

2 teaspoons garlic salt

1 teaspoon ground ginger

1/2 teaspoon oregano

2 teaspoons paprika

1/2 teaspoon thyme

vegetable or canola oil for frying

ranch for serving

hot sauce for serving

ketchup for serving

INSTRUCTIONS

In a large bowl, whisk together the buttermilk, hot sauce, fresh thyme, 1 teaspoon salt, and 1 teaspoon black pepper.

Slice the potatoes into 1/4-inch to 1/2-inch thick rounds and place into the seasoned buttermilk. Give them a toss to coat evenly in the buttermilk. Cover with plastic wrap and chill for at least 30 minutes or up to 2 hours! You don't want anything longer than that or else they'll begin to turn brown.

In a separate bowl, combine the flour, remaining salt, remaining pepper, and the rest of the spices until evenly incorporated. Add in about 3 tablespoons of the buttermilk from the potatoes and toss until coarse crumbs are formed.
Working with a few potato slices at a time, carefully remove from the buttermilk (allowing excess to drip off) and place into the seasoned flour. Toss around until evenly coated, and then place on a baking sheet. Continue coating the remaining potatoes until they're all done. Allow to air dry for about 10 minutes to ensure the coating sticks to the potatoes.

Meanwhile, fill a large, heavy-bottom pan, about halfway with oil. Set a candy thermometer in and heat over medium-high until the temperature reaches 365 degrees F. Once hot, carefully drop in a few potatoes at a time and fry until golden brown and crispy on both sides, about 3 to 4 minutes. Remove from a slotted spoon onto a wire rack set over a baking sheet. Keep warm in a preheated 200 degree F oven while you continue frying the rest. As soon as the potatoes come out of the oil, season lightly with salt.

Serve the potatoes with ranch, ketchup and hot sauce on the side and a sprinkling of fresh thyme.
Enjoy!

VEGAN ARTICHOKE DIP

PREP TIME: 15minutes
TOTAL TIME: 15minutes
SERVINGS: 4
CALORIES: 295 kcal

INGREDIENTS

1 jar (12 oz / 340 g) oil-packed marinated artichoke hearts
1 can (14 oz / 400 g) white beans, drained and rinsed
½ teaspoon garlic powder
½ teaspoon onion powder
½ teaspoon salt
2 - 3 tablespoons of oil from the jar of marinated artichoke hearts
Optional for garnish: your favorite herb additional chopped artichoke hearts, an extra drizzle of oil.

INSTRUCTIONS

Drain the jar of artichoke hearts, reserving the oil. Roughly chop the hearts into smallish chunks (like what you'd find in a dip).
Place the beans, half of the chopped artichoke hearts, garlic and onion powder, salt and 2 tablespoons of the oil in a small food processor. Blend until totally smooth.

If you want it a bit thinner, add another tablespoon of oil. Taste and adjust the seasonings if necessary.

Transfer to a bowl and stir in the other half of the chopped artichoke hearts.
Garnish as desired and serve with your favorite dipper

ORIGINAL AVOCADO SALAD

SERVINGS: 6
PREP 15 Minutes
READY IN: 15minutes

INGREDIENTS

1 medium (12 oz) English cucumber, cut into quarters through the length then sliced
16 oz. grape tomatoes
1/2 small red onion,sliced into small pieces
2 medium avocados (firm but ripe), sliced into bite size pieces

DRESSING

1 1/2 Tbsp fresh lemon juice
1 1/2 Tbsp red wine vinegar
3 1/2 Tbsp extra virgin olive oil
1 tsp honey
1 1/2 tsp minced garlic
1/4 cup chopped cilantro
1/4 cup chopped parsley
1/2 tsp dried oregano
Salt and freshly ground black pepper

INSTRUCTIONS

For the dressing: In a small mixing bowl whisk together lemon juice, red wine vinegar, extra virgin oil oil, honey, garlic, cilantro, parsley, oregano, and season with salt and pepper to taste.

In a large bowl gently toss together cucumbers, tomatoes, red onion, and avocado with dressing.

Serve shortly after preparing.

NOTES

I like to use a multicolor blend of tomatoes for a more visually appealing salad but all red tomatoes work just fine too.

BLACK BEANS HUMMUS

PREP TIME: 5 mins
TOTAL TIME: 5 mins
SERVINGS: 8

INGREDIENTS

1 (15 ounce) can black beans

1 clove garlic

2 tablespoons lemon juice, or more to taste

1 1/2 tablespoons tahini

1/2 teaspoon ground cumin, or more to taste

1/2 teaspoon salt, or more to taste

1/8 teaspoon cayenne pepper, or more to taste

1/4 teaspoon paprika, or as needed

10 Greek olives

INSTRUCTION

Drain beans and reserve liquid.

Place garlic into the bowl of a food processor and pulse until minced. Add black beans, 2 tablespoons bean

liquid, lemon juice, tahini, cumin, salt, and cayenne pepper; process until smooth, scraping down the sides as needed.
Taste and add additional bean liquid, lemon juice, tahini, cumin, salt, and cayenne pepper as needed. Transfer to a serving bowl and sprinkle with paprika. Arrange Greek olives over top.

MELON AND WATERCRESS SALAD

TOTAL TIME: 15 minutes
 YIELD: 4 servings

INGREDIENTS

2 tablespoons lemon juice
¼ teaspoon Celtic sea salt
1 tablespoon raw honey
2 tablespoons extra virgin olive oil
3 cups watercress chopped
3 cups watermelon cubes
1 cup seedless cucumber cut into cubes
2 radishes sliced into thin rounds
15 fresh basil leaves cut into ribbons or chopped
½ cup crumbled feta cheese chopped or ¼ cup tamari roasted sunflower seeds (optional)

INSTRUCTIONS

In a small bowl whisk together the lemon juice, salt and honey until dissolved. Whisk in the olive oil until emulsified. Set aside.

Place the watercress, watermelon, cucumbers, radishes and basil in a large bowl.

Drizzle with enough vinaigrette to coat the watercress lightly and toss well. Taste for seasonings and serve immediately.

Serve on 4 individual plates topped with feta cheese or sunflower seeds.

Enjoy immediately.

CHAPTER 4 : RED MEAT
Grilled spiced chops

READY IN: 1 hr 40 mins
SERVES: 4

INGREDIENTS

1/3 teaspoon ground ginger

1/4 teaspoon allspice

1 teaspoon curry powder

1 teaspoon oregano

1 cup tomato sauce

3 tablespoons cider vinegar

3 garlic cloves, smashed and chopped

1/4 teaspoon cayenne pepper (optional)

 salt, to taste

 black pepper, to taste

8 lamb chops, trimmed of fat (2.5 cm thick)

INSTRUCTION

place all ingredients, except lamb chops in sauce pan. boil 10 minutes.

place lamb chops in deep glass dish and pour sauce over them. marinate 1 hour.

preheat barbecue at med-high.

oil grill and add lamb chops. cover and cook 6 to 7 minutes on each side. after meat is seared, season well and baste with marinade during cooking.

BEEF STUFFED ZUCCHINI

READY IN: 25 mins
SERVES: 4
YIELDS: 4 zucchini shells

INGREDIENTS

4 medium zucchini
1 lb lean ground beef
1/2 cup sweet onion, chopped
1 egg
3/4 cup marinara sauce
1/4 cup seasoned bread crumbs
 salt and pepper (to taste and dietary needs)
1 cup monterey jack cheese, shredded, divided
1 cup marinara sauce, for serving

INSTRUCTION

Cut zucchini in half lengthwise; cut a thin slice from the bottom of each so they sit flat. Scoop out pulp, leaving a 1/4 inch shell.

Place shells in an ungreased 13x9 microwave safe dish (or any size that will fit all four pieces - mine is round). Turn off turntable setting on microwave (I remove the turntable).

Cover dish and microwave on HIGH for 3 minutes or until crisp tender; drain and set aside.

In a large skillet, cook beef and onion over medium heat until meat is no longer pink and broken up well; drain.

Remove skillet from heat and stir in egg, marinara sauce, bread crumbs, salt, pepper and 1/2 cup cheese.

Spoon about a 1/4 cup into each shell. Microwave, uncovered, on HIGH for 4 minutes.
Sprinkle with remaining 1/2 cup cheese then microwave for 3-4 minutes longer until therm
ometer inserted into filling read 160°F.
Serve with warmed up marinara sauce for each serving for dipping.

PURELY SPANISH PORK CUTLETS AND ONIONS

PREP 10min
COOK 10min

INGREDIENTS

Pork loin fillets 4
Manchego cheese 4 slices
Quince jelly 4 slices
Olive oil
Salt & pepper
Flour
Beaten egg
Breadcrumbs
Tomatoes, black olives, onions for garnish
Lemon wedges 4

INSTRUCTION

Thinly the slice the cheese and quince jelly to match the size of the pork.

Score the pork loins before slicing into half horizontally or score to make a pocket.

Fill the pork loin with the sliced cheese and jelly.

Season the stuffed pork with salt & pepper, dredge with flour, dip in the beaten egg and cover liberally with the breadcrumbs. Deep fry at 170C.

In the meantime, cut the tomatoes into wedges, cut the olives into half, finely chop the onions and mix well.

Add olive oil, salt & pepper to Step 5 to make a salad.

Arrange the fried pork and salad onto a serving dish with the lemon wedges.

Quince jelly is made from marmelo and goes really well with Manchego cheese.

Manchego cheese is a hard Spanish sheep's cheese

GARLIC AND BACON PLATTER

YIELD 4 serving(s)
PREP TIME 30 Min
COOK TIME 30 Min
METHOD Stove Top

INGREDIENTS
60 little neck clams
8 strips of bacon, sliced
1 sm onions, small white, chopped
1 stalk celery, chopped
6 baby carrots, chopped small
1 c white wine
1/2 stick butter
12 oz soba noodles
10 clove garlic peeled
crusty bread of choice
1 can diced tomatoes

INSTRUCTION
Gather your goods!! Put your clams in a large bowl or pot under cold running water, remove surface dirt and debris, then fill container with water so the clams will release extra grit and sand.
Wash and prep your other veggies. Get pot of water on for noodles. I prefer the green tea noodles or buck wheat. They are light and flavorful, beautiful with this dish. Prepare according to package. Boil about 6 minutes, drain and set a side

While noodles are being prepared, take the cut up bacon and saute in large pot over medium high heat. After bacon begins to render add veggies continue to cook until bacon is crisping. Add garlic, and cook till garlic aroma fills the air. Add wine and tomatoes bring to boil.

Rinse clams again, drain and add to the bacon / veggie mix. cook until clams open. As the open, move them out of pan to make room for more clams as they open.

Meal while, toast your bread of choice, however is best for you, I prefer the grill, but an oven is perfect.

Now that your clams are all open, place the soba noodles in the remaining broth and add the butter. stir around, return clams to broth, add more wine if needed. Serve on a large platter with crusty bread.

Enjoy and have fun with your guest. Put any remaining broth in a few side cups for your guest, just in case they want more!

CHAPTER 5 : DESSERT
Fine baked apple

PREP TIME: 15 minutes
COOK TIME: 45 minutes
TOTAL TIME: 1 hour
YIELD: 4

INGREDIENTS

3 Tablespoons (43g) unsalted butter, softened to room temperature (extra soft, so it's easy to mash)
1/4 cup (50g) packed light or dark brown sugar
1/2 teaspoon ground cinnamon
1/8 teaspoon ground nutmeg
1/4 cup (21g) old-fashioned whole rolled oats
4 large apples (see note), rinsed and patted dry
optional: 2 Tablespoons raisins, dried cranberries, or chopped nuts

FOR BAKING

3/4 cup (180ml) warm water
INSTRUCTIONS
Preheat oven to 375°F (191°C).

Using a handheld or stand mixer with a paddle attachment, or simply using a fork or spoon, beat/mash the butter, sugar, cinnamon, and nutmeg together until combined. Stir in the oats, then the raisins/dried cranberries/nuts, if using. Set aside.

Core the apples: This can be tricky, but I recommend using a sharp paring knife and a spoon. (Or an apple corer.) I find cookie scoops can easily break or crack the apples. Using a sharp paring knife, cut around the core, about halfway or 3/4 down into the apple. Use a spoon to carefully dig out the core. Takes a bit of patience and arm muscle. Once the core is out, use a spoon to dig out any more seeds.

Place cored apples in an 8-inch or 9-inch baking pan, cake pan, or pie dish. Spoon filling into each apple, filling all the way to the top. Pour warm water into the pan around the apples. The water helps prevent the apples from drying out and burning.

Bake for 40-45 minutes or until apples appear slightly soft. Bake longer for softer, mushier baked apples. The time depends on how firm your apples were and how soft you want them to be.

Remove apples from the oven and, if desired, baste the outside of the apples with juices from the pan. This adds a little moisture to the skin, but it's completely optional.

Serve warm with salted caramel, whipped cream, or ice cream. Cover and store leftovers in the refrigerator for up to 2 days.

COOL CARROT BALL

TOTAL TIME: 55 mins
YIELD: 25-30 balls

INGREDIENTS

300 g/10.5 oz grated carrots (about 3 cups)
100 g/3.5 oz oats (about 1 cup)
2 tbsp ground flaxseed
1 onion, chopped
3 cloves of garlic, minced
1 tbsp mustard
1 tbsp tomato paste or ketchup
1.5 tsp paprika powder
1 tsp curry powder
1/2 tsp chili powder
2–3 tbsp bread crumbs (use GF if needed)
salt, pepper

INSTRUCTIONS

Start by preparing flax egg: in a small bowl whisk together ground flaxseeds with about 8 tablespoons of water. Let rest for 5 minutes to thicken.

Add flax egg and rest of the ingredients to a large bowl and mix well together. If you prefer a smoother finish, you can also add the mixture to a food processor and pulse a few times. Adjust seasoning if needed, then cover and let rest for 30 minutes.

Meanwhile preheat the oven to 200°C/400°F. Form mixture into small balls with wet hands (use about 2 tablespoons of mixture per ball), and place them on a baking sheet. Bake for 15-20 minutes on each side or until golden brown.

Alternatively, fry them in hot oil until crispy, about 3-3 minutes each side.

Enjoy!

PUMPKIN CAKE MUFFINS

PREP TIME: 15 minutes
 COOK TIME: 21 minutes
 TOTAL Time: 45 minutes
 YIELD: 12 muffins

INGREDIENTS

1 and 3/4 cups (219g) all-purpose flour (spooned & leveled)
1 teaspoon baking soda
1 and 1/2 teaspoons ground cinnamon
1 and 1/2 teaspoons pumpkin pie spice*
1/4 teaspoon ground ginger
1/2 teaspoon salt
1/2 cup (120ml) vegetable oil (or melted coconut oil)
1/2 cup (100g) granulated sugar
1/3 cup (67g) packed light or dark brown sugar
1 and 1/2 cups (340g) canned pumpkin puree (not pumpkin pie filling)
2 large eggs
1/4 cup (60ml) milk (dairy or nondairy)

INSTRUCTIONS

Preheat oven to 425°F (218°C). Spray a 12-count muffin pan with nonstick spray or line with cupcake liners.
In a large bowl, whisk the flour, baking soda, cinnamon, pumpkin pie spice, ginger, and salt together until combined. Set aside.
In a medium bowl, whisk the oil, granulated sugar, brown sugar, pumpkin puree, eggs, and milk together

until combined. Pour the wet ingredients into the dry ingredients, and then fold everything together gently just until combined and no flour pockets remain.

Spoon the batter into liners, filling them all the way to the top.

Bake for 5 minutes at 425°F, then, keeping the muffins in the oven, reduce the oven temperature to 350°F (177°C). Bake for an additional 16–17 minutes or until a toothpick inserted in the center comes out clean. The total time these muffins take in the oven is about 21–22 minutes, give or take. Allow the muffins to cool for 5 minutes in the muffin pan before enjoying.

Cover tightly and store at room temperature for up to 1 week.

APPLE SAUCE BEAN BROWNIES

INGREDIENTS

1- 15 oz can black beans, rinsed and brain

2 eggs

1/2 cup unsweetened applesauce

1/2 cup coconut sugar

5 tbsp cocoa powder

1 tsp baking powder

1/8 tsp salt

1 tsp vanilla

OPTIONAL:

You can add semi chocolate chips or nuts

INSTRUCTION

1. Preheat oven to 350 degrees

2. Add all ingredients to a food processor and mix until all ingredients are well blended

3. Spray an 8×8 baking dish with non stick cooking spray

4. Pour batter into pan. If adding chocolate chips or nuts, add on top.

5. Bake for 25 minutes until toothpick comes out clean after inserting into the centre

6. Cool for 30 minutes, cut and serve

HEALTHY BEANS BALL

PREP:15 mins
COOK:15 mins
SERVINGS:12

INGREDIENTS

1 x 400 g can no-added-salt chickpeas, drained
1/2 cup frozen peas, defrosted
1/2 cup carrot, sweet potato or pumpkin, grated
1/2 onion, finely chopped
1 clove garlic, finely chopped
3 tbs wholemeal plain flour
1 tbs sweet chilli sauce
1 tsp ground cumin, optional
1 tsp ground coriander, optional
1 tbs canola oil

INGREDIENTS

Mash the chickpeas and peas together in a large bowl with a fork or potato masher.
With your hands, squeeze as much moisture as you can out of the grated vegetables and add them the bowl.
Add all the other ingredients (except the oil) and mix well.
Take a big spoonful of the mixture and roll into a ball with your hands. Flatten the ball and place on a plate. Repeat with the rest of the mixture.
Heat half the oil in a large, non-stick frying pan. Add about half the balls, being careful not to overcrowd the

pan. Cook for 2-3 minutes, until golden brown, then flip over and cook for another 2-3 minutes. Place them on paper towel while you cook the rest of the balls.

NOTE

If you have a food processor or stick blender with a bowl attachment, add all the ingredients (except the oil) to the food processor and blitz till you get a chunky but sticky texture. Then continue from step 4.

CHAPTER 6 : CHICKEN AND POULTRY RECIPE

Roasted tomatoes soup

PREP TIME: 15 MINUTES
COOK TIME: 30 MINUTES
TOTAL TIME: 45 MINUTES
YIELD: 4 TO 6 Servings

INGREDIENT

3 1/2 pounds ripe tomatoes (any small- to medium-sized tomatoes will do)
3 tablespoons olive oil, divided
fine sea salt and freshly-cracked black pepper
1 large white or yellow onion, diced
5 cloves garlic, minced
3/4 teaspoon smoked paprika
1/4 teaspoon crushed red pepper flakes
2 1/2 cups vegetable broth
1/2 cup loosely-packed fresh basil leaves
optional toppings: freshly-grated Parmesan, drizzle of heavy cream or olive oil, croutons, sour cream or fresh basil

INSTRUCTIONS

Roast the tomatoes. Heat oven to 450°F. Quarter the tomatoes (or halve them, if they are small) and arrange them cut-side-up on a baking sheet. Drizzle evenly with 2 tablespoons of the olive oil and season with a few pinches of salt and black pepper. Bake for 30 to 40 minutes or until softened, then transfer baking sheet to a wire rack.

Sauté the onion and garlic. Meanwhile, heat the remaining 1 tablespoon of olive oil in a large stockpot over medium-high heat. Add the onion and sauté for 5 minutes, stirring occasionally. Add the garlic, smoked paprika and crushed red pepper flakes and sauté for 2 more minutes, stirring frequently.

Put it all together. Add the broth, basil, and the roasted tomatoes (once they are ready) with their juices and stir to combine.

Purée. Using a handheld immersion blender (or see instructions below for using a traditional blender), purée the soup until it reaches your desired texture.

Season. Taste the soup and season with extra salt, pepper, and/or smoked paprika as needed.

Serve. Serve warm, garnished with any extra toppings you would like, and

enjoy!

EPIC MANGO CHICKEN

Cooking Time: 20 min
SERVINGS : 4

INGREDIENTS

1 lime
2 tbsp Mango Lassi Mix
2 tbsp olive oil
1 tbsp low sodium soy sauce
1 lb (450 g) boneless, skinless chicken thighs
2 red bell peppers
1 green bell pepper
2 cups frozen mango chunks
Toppings (optional): Everything Bagel Whole Food Topper, sliced green onion

INSTRUCTION

Preheat oven to 450° F. Line Sheet Pan with Sheet Pan Liner.

Cut lime in half. In a large bowl, using 2-in-1 Citrus Press, squeeze in juice from lime. Stir in mix, olive oil, and soy sauce to make glaze. Toss chicken in glaze, set aside.

Slice bell peppers. Add bell peppers and mango to glaze; toss to coat.

Arrange evenly on pan. Cook 16–18 min or until chicken is cooked through. Add toppings, if desired.

SOY TURKEY MEAT BALL

INGREDIENTS

Meatballs

1 kg ground turkey or half turkey half pork, or other meat

1 small onion chopped

4 cloves garlic minced

1 bunch coriander finely chopped

2 egg yolks (or 1 egg +1 yolk, I just reserve the egg whites for baking)

2 tsp white pepper

1 tbsp salt

1 tbsp miso paste

2 tbsp gochujang can sub for other chili pastes

3 tbsp cold water* or stock

1 1/2 tbsp dried herbs optional

Few drops of sesame oil optional

Oil for frying as needed

Glaze

60 g maple syrup around 1/4 cup

120 ml soy sauce around 1/2 cup

INSTRUCTIONS

Mix everything together for the meatballs except for the oil until everything is homogeneous. Don't over-mix as they will start to get tough.

Make meatballs by scooping out about a tablespoon of the mixture and rolling it into a smooth ball. You can do all of this in advance before you turn the stove on and leave them on a tray or in the mixing bowl so they're ready for you to cook. Or just roll them as you go but that's messier.

Heat a large pan over medium heat with enough oil to cover the bottom. Cook the meatballs, turning them to brown on all sides until fully cooked, around 7 min.** Set aside.

In a small sauce pan, add maple syrup and soy sauce and cook on medium high until bubbling. Whisk frequently so it doesn't burn, take off the heat once it thickens enough to coat the back of a spoon. Make sure to taste it around half way through the thickening process and at the end, as the sugars will caramelize and it will be a lot different from when you first poured the mix in.

Pour the glaze over the meatballs and toss/stir to coat evenly.

Enjoy!

NOTES

Adding water helps keep the meatballs juicy & tender! This is also done when making dumpling filling.

No harming in splitting open a few to make sure they're cooked, keep them small if you're worried they won't cook through fully.

ORANGE PINEAPPLE CHICKEN

YIELD MAKES: 4 servings
PREP TIME 15 min.
COOK TIME 15 min.

INGREDIENTS

1 can (20 oz.) Pineapple Chunks, drained, juice reserved
2 cups Brown Rice, uncooked
1 lb. chicken breast, cut into 1/2-inch pieces
2 tablespoons all-purpose flour
1 tablespoon vegetable oil
1 cup red bell pepper, chopped
1 cup sugar snap peas
2/3 cup Sweet and Sour Sauce
1/4 cup Reduced Sodium Soy Sauce
1 large orange, zested and juiced or 1/2 cup fresh orange juice
1/2 teaspoon crushed red chilies, optional
1/4 cup toasted chopped cashews
Sliced green onions, optional

INSTRUCTION

Measure reserved pineapple juice and add enough water to make 1-3/4 cups liquid. Prepare rice according to package directions using juice-water mixture. Coat chicken pieces with flour.

Heat oil in large skillet or wok over medium-high heat and cook chicken until edges are golden brown, about 5

to 7 minutes. Add pineapple, bell pepper and snap
peas. Cook until slightly softened, about 3 minutes.
Add sweet and sour sauce, soy sauce, orange juice and
red chilies, if desired to pan. Stir and cook an additional
3 minutes or until sauce begins to boil. Stir in orange
zest. Serve over rice topped with cashews and green
onions

CHICKEN MUSHROOMS MEATBALL

PREP TIME: 20minutes
COOK TIME: 22minutes
TOTAL TIME: 42 minutes

INGREDIENTS
For the chicken meatballs mix
1 pound Chicken meat minced
½ cup Parsley minced
1 cup Mushroom chopped
½ cup Parmesan
½ cup Scamorza (see notes)
⅓ cup Breadcrumbs
1 pinch Salt
1 pinch Black Pepper crushed
For the cooking sauce
2 cups Mushrooms sliced
3 tsp Garlic minced
1 tbsp Olive oil extra virgin
⅓ cup Cream
2 tbsp Parsley chopped

INSTRUCTIONS
Make the meatballs
Add in a bowl all the ingredients to mix the chicken meatballs.

Mix all the ingredients until they are evenly combined.

Scoop 1 and a 1/2 tablespoon of the mix and shape the mix into a ball of around 2 inches diameter.

Place the meatballs on a chopping board or a plate and set aside until you will cook them (see notes).

Cook the chicken meatballs with mushrooms

Heat 1 tbsp of evoo in a frying pan.

When the oil shimmers, add the garlic minced and cook it for 2 minutes.

Add the sliced mushrooms and cook them for 5 minutes.

Add the chicken meatballs and cook them until they are done for 10-12 minutes on low-to-medium heat.

Add the cream and keep on cooking for few more minutes.

Plate the meatballs, sprinkle the parsley and MANGIA!

NOTES

You can sub the scamorza with provolone cheese.

You can make the meatballs in advance and keep them in the refrigerator for 24 hours until you are ready to cook them.

This recipe is freezable, you can in fact freeze it in portions in a zip-bag for 6 weeks. To reheat the balls, just remove them from the freezer and thaw them overnight in the refrigerator, warming them up in a buttered frying pan

BBQ TURKEY MEATBALL

PREP TIME: 10 mins
COOK TIME: 30 mins
TOTAL TIME: 40 mins
SERVES: 4

INGREDIENTS
1- 1.5 pounds ground turkey
½ cup onion, very finely minced
1 egg
¼ cup breadcrumbs
1 teaspoon garlic powder
1 teaspoon chili powder
½ teaspoon paprika
½ teaspoon kosher salt
¾ cup BBQ sauce, divided
2 tablespoons oil

INSTRUCTIONS
Preheat the oven to 375. Line a baking sheet with parchment paper (not totally required but makes for much easier cleanup!).

In a large bowl, using your hands, mix together all the ingredients except the BBQ sauce and oil.

Mix in 3-4 tablespoons of the BBQ sauce; enough to help it bind and add flavor. If you feel like your mixture is too moist add more breadcrumbs.

Heat the oil in the skillet.

Roll the turkey mixture into 1½ inch balls and drop into the heated skillet in batches (I cook about 8 at a time)

Roll them around after a minute so they brown relatively evenly. Remove the browned meatballs to the prepared baking sheet and repeat until they are all browned.

Spoon the remaining BBQ sauce over each meatball and bake for 15-20 minutes, until they are cooked through.

Serve with more BBQ sauce if you're feeling saucy.

NOTES

I usually get about 36 meatballs from this recipe.

CHAPTER 7 : BEEF AND PORK RECIPE

Roasted toco wraps

PREP TIME: 5 minutes
COOK TIME: 15 minutes
TOTAL TIME: 20 minutes

INGREDIENTS

1 pound ground beef
1 sweet onion, peeled and chopped
1/2 cup taco sauce (as spicy as you like!)
1 cup shredded cheddar or Jack cheese, or a combo of both
4 flour tortillas (8 inch tacos work best, size-wise)
Any of the following as garnish: chopped iceberg lettuce, sour cream, guacamole, salsa, etc!

INSTRUCTIONS

Saute ground beef and onion in a medium skillet over medium high heat until beef is brown and onion is tender. Stir in taco sauce until heated through.

Heat the tortillas by either putting them in the microwave for about 20 seconds, or by wrapping them in foil and heating them in a conventional oven for about 15 minutes at 375.

Assemble as follows: divide the meat mixture among the tortillas, placing it at the bottom third of the tortilla. Top with cheese and your choice of garnish. Starting with the filling end of the tortilla, slowly roll it up, tucking the side ends in towards the center if you like. Cut in half and serve at once.

NOTES

Tortillas: Make sure you use flour tortillas for this recipe, as corn tortillas are not as flexible and may break when they are folded. I use 8 inch size tortillas.

Spice Level: This all depends on how spicy your taco sauce is. I like mild, but I am a big old spice wimp, so if you like more heat, use regular or spicy taco sauce and you are all set.

BEEF BROCCOLI DINNER

PREP: 15 minutes
COOK: 18 minutes
TOTAL: 33 minutes

INGREDIENTS

1 lb. beef sliced into thin pieces
2 cups broccoli cut into florets
2 teaspoons ginger minced
2 cloves garlic minced
1 tablespoon cornstarch
1/2 to 3/4 cups water optional
¼ cup cooking oil
Salt and ground black pepper to taste

MARINADE INGREDIENTS:

1/4 cup oyster sauce
1 tablespoon Knorr Liquid Seasoning
1/2 teaspoon Sesame oil optional
3 tablespoons cooking wine optional
1 teaspoon granulated white sugar

INSTRUCTIONS

Combine beef, oyster sauce, Knorr Liquid Seasoning, Sesame oil, cooking wine, and sugar in a bowl. Mix well. Marinate beef for 15 minutes. Add cornstarch and mix to blend with all the ingredients. Set aside.
Heat 2 tablespoons cooking oil in a cooking pot. Sauté ginger and garlic. Add broccoli before the garlic starts to

brown. Stir-fry for 1 to 2 minutes. Remove from the pot. Set aside.

Pour the remaining oil into the pot. Add marinated beef once the oil gets hot. Stir-fry until the beef browns. You can add water to tenderize the beef further. If water is added, let it boil and stir as it evaporates. Add salt and ground black pepper to taste.

Put the cooked broccoli into the pot with the beef. Stir-fry for 3 minutes.

Transfer to a serving plate.

Serve

BEEF PENNE MEAL

PREP: 5 mins
COOK: 1 hr 10 mins
TOTAL: 1 hr 15 mins
SERVES: 5

INGREDIENTS

¾ lb penne pasta, cooked & cooled
2 lb beef short ribs, boneless, cut into 1½-inch cubes
7 oz bacon rashers, or pancetta, diced
6 oz celery, diced
5½ oz red onions, diced
3 oz carrots, diced
6 cloves garlic, minced or grated
1⅓ lb marinara sauce
1 cup red wine
1¼ cups beef broth
4 tbsp tomato paste
1½ tbsp olive oil
1¼ tbsp Italian seasoning
2 pcs bay leaves
2 tsp brown sugar
salt and ground black pepper, to season and taste

To Serve:

⅛ tsp parsley, per serving
½ tsp parmesan cheese, per serving

INSTRUCTIONS

Heat up the oil in a deep skillet or Dutch oven over medium-high heat.

Add your beef and sear evenly on all sides, roughly 3 minutes on each side.

Add bacon or pancetta and saute until crispy, roughly 6 to 8 minutes. Set aside.

Add onions, celery, carrots, and Italian seasoning into the same Dutch oven with bacon fat. Saute until translucent.

Add garlic and tomato paste. Roast briefly.

Deglaze with red wine and reduce briefly.

Add sugar, beef broth, bay leaves, and marinara sauce. Mix to combine and bring to a boil.

Add the beef and bacon back into the pot and reduce heat to medium. Cover and simmer for roughly 40 minutes or until beef are fork-tender.

Discard the bay leaves and add your pasta while your sauce is still hot. Mix until evenly incorporated.

Season with salt and pepper. Adjust accordingly.

Portion accordingly. Serve with parmesan cheese and garnish with parsley or basil.

MUSTARD LAMB CUTLETS

COOKING TIME: less than 15 minutes
SERVES: 4

INGREDIENTS

80ml (1/3 cup) olive oil
2 tablespoons Dijon mustard
1 tablespoon chopped fresh parsley
2 tablespoons soy sauce
6 cloves garlic, crushed
freshly ground black pepper
12 lamb cutlets

INSTRUCTION

Place oil, mustard, parsley, sauce, garlic and pepper in medium bowl; whisk until combined.
Trim fat from cutlets. Coat cutlets with mustard mixture. Cook lamb, in batches, on heated, oiled griddle (or grill, or barbecue) until browned on both sides and cooked as desired.
Serve lamb with roast potatoes and steamed asparagus, if desired.

Uncooked lamb suitable to freeze.
Not suitable to microwave.

CHAPTER 8 : FISH AND SEAFOOD

Classic crab cakes

TOTAL TIME: 25 mins
SERVINGS: 4

INGREDIENTS

⅔ cup panko (Japanese breadcrumbs), divided
1 tablespoon minced fresh flat-leaf parsley
2 tablespoons finely chopped green onions
2 tablespoons canola mayonnaise
1 teaspoon lemon juice
1 teaspoon Dijon mustard
½ teaspoon Old Bay seasoning
½ teaspoon Worcestershire sauce
⅛ teaspoon kosher salt
⅛ teaspoon ground red pepper
1 large egg, lightly beaten
8 ounces lump crabmeat, shell pieces removed
1 tablespoon olive oil
1 lemon, quartered

INSTRUCTION

Combine 1/3 cup panko, parsley, green onion, mayonnaise, lemon juice mustard, Old Bay seasoning, Worcestershire, salt, pepper and egg in a large bowl, stirring well. Add crab; stir gently just until combined. Place remaining 1/3 cup panko in a shallow dish. Using wet hands, shape crab mixture into 4 equal balls. Coat balls in the remaining panko. Gently flatten balls to form 4 (4-inch) patties.

Heat a large nonstick skillet over medium-high heat. Add oil to pan; swirl to coat. Add patties; cook 3 minutes on each side or until golden. Serve with lemon wedges.

Variation to Try
Prepare Classic Crab Cakes recipe, substituting 8 ounces cooked, flaked salmon for the crab. Serves 4 (serving size: 1 salmon cake and 1 lemon wedge) calories 210; fat 11 g (sat 4g); sodium 307mg

NO-FUSS TUNA SALAD

YIELD: 6 sandwiches
PREP TIME: 10 minutes
 TOTAL TIME: 10 minutes

INGREDIENTS

3 cans (5 oz. each) tuna in water, drained
1 stalk of celery, finely chopped
half of a medium onion, finely chopped
1/2 cup mayonnaise
2 tablespoons sweet pickle relish
salt and pepper, to taste
bread slices, toasted if you prefer
lettuce, tomatoes, other toppings (optional)

INSTRUCTIONS

In a medium bowl, combine the tuna, celery, onion, mayonnaise, parsley, pickle relish, salt, and pepper. Taste and adjust the seasonings if necessary.
Top one bread/toast slice with some of the tuna mixture. Spread mixture evenly. Add lettuce, tomato, etc., if desired. Top with another bread/toast slice. Cut in half if desired.

Serve immediately.

NOTES

I'm often asked about the addition of eggs. Feel free to add a couple of chopped hard-boiled eggs to the tuna mixture if you like it that way! Depending on the consistency you like, you may need to add a tad more mayo.

Not a fan of sweet pickle relish? Try dill relish - or omit it entirely.

I love adding fresh herbs to my tuna salad when I have fresh herbs on hand. Thyme, basil, dill, and parsley are all great.

Want to change it up a bit? Try adding some Cajun seasoning ... it's awesome!

Refrigerate leftovers in an airtight container for up to 3-5 days.

SHRIMP GREEN CURRY

PREP TIME: 20 minutes
COOK TIME: 15 Minutes
TOTAL TIME: 35 minutes
YIELD: serves 4

INGREDIENTS
GREEN CURRY PASTE:
3 green chiles (like jalapeno or serrano) roughly chopped
1/4 cup cilantro leaves
2 lemongrass stems, trim and use only bottom 4 inches (If using frozen chopped, use 3 tablespoons)
2 Tablespoons chopped galangal
5 cloves garlic
2 tablespoons dried shrimp, soaked in hot water for 15 minutes (use miso for vegetarians or omit entirely)
1 tablespoon peeled and roughly chopped ginger
2 large shallots, peeled and roughly chopped
4 large kaffir lime leaves
2 Tablespoons fish sauce (use 2 Tablespoons water and 1 teaspoon salt if vegetarian)
1 teaspoon ground cumin
1 teaspoon ground coriander
¼ teaspoon ground turmeric
¼ teaspoon ground black pepper
4 Tablespoons light brown sugar
GREEN CURRY SHRIMP
3 tablespoons neutral oil
6 tablespoons green curry paste, divided

2 large cloves garlic minced
1 Tablespoon peeled and minced ginger
1 ½ lb large shrimp (21-25 size)
1 can coconut milk (12-13 oz)
3 Tablespoons fish sauce
1 medium chinese eggplant
½ large onion, thinly sliced
6 oz shiitake mushrooms
1 ½ oz baby spinach (large handful)
FOR SERVING
Hot rice
Limes Wedges

INSTRUCTIONS
MAKE THE CURRY PASTE:
Drain the dried shrimp.

Place the dried shrimp, chilis, cilantro, lemongrass, galangal, garlic, dried shrimp, ginger, shallots, kaffir limes leaves, fish sauce, cumin, turmeric, coriander, black pepper, and brown sugar in a food processor or blender and process until smooth, about 1 minute. (If you're having problems blending, add a tablespoon or two of water).

Set aside or refrigerate until ready to make the curry. (You will only use about ⅓ of the paste. You can split and then freeze the remaining paste to use for future curries.)

Prepare Green Shrimp Curry:

Trim the stem off of the eggplant and then cut it into ½ inch pieces. (I used a roll cut where you turn the eggplant a ¼ turn after each cut. But you can just cut it into rounds.) Set aside.

Trim the hard stems off of the shiitakes and discard. Cut the mushrooms into thick slices. Set aside.

Heat a frying pan over medium heat and add the oil and 2 Tablespoons of the spice paste. Stir-fry for 1 minute until fragrant. Add the onions and stir fry for 2-3 minutes. (The paste may start to brown and stick to the bottom of the pan, but just keep scraping and stirring.)

Add the ginger, garlic, eggplant and mushrooms and stir fry for another minute. Add the coconut milk, 4 more tablespoons of green curry paste, and 3 Tablespoons of fish sauce.

Bring the mixture to a simmer. Stir, scraping the bottom and sides of the pan.

Lower heat to medium, cover the pot with a lid, and cook for 4-5 minutes until the eggplant has softened.

Add the shrimp and cook for 2-3 minutes. Taste and adjust seasoning with a little salt or fish sauce as needed.

Add the spinach and stir to wilt.

Serve immediately with hot rice and lime wedges.

SALMON PEAS MEAL

INGREDIENTS

240g wholewheat fusilli
knob of butter
1 large shallot, finely chopped
140g frozen peas
2 skinless salmon filets, cut into chunks
140g low-fat crème fraîche
½ low-salt vegetable stock cube
small bunch of chives, snipped

INSTRUCTION

Bring a pan of water to the boil and cook the fusilli according to the pack instructions.

Meanwhile, heat a knob of butter in a saucepan, then add the shallot and cook for 5 mins or until softened.

Add the peas, salmon, crème fraîche and 50 ml water. Crumble in the stock cube.

Cook for 3-4 mins until cooked through, stir in the chives and some black pepper. Then stir through to coat the pasta. Serve in bowls.

LOVELY MEDITERRANEAN FISH

PREP TIME 5 minutes mins
COOK TIME 25 minutes mins
TOTAL TIME 32 minutes mins
SERVING 6 people

INGREDIENTS

2 1/2 lbs cod, or another firm white fish cut in 6-7 oz pieces
white or yellow onion cut in half then sliced
8 garlic cloves sliced
2 tbsp olive oil extra virgin
28 oz crushed tomatoes
1/2 cup chicken broth
10-12 oz small vine cherry tomatoes sub out for a pint of grape tomatoes
3 oz kalamata olives
5 oz castelvetrano olives
3 tbsp fresh parsley minced
1 tbsp fresh oregano or 1 tsp dried oregano

INSTRUCTIONS

If the cod isn't already pre butchered, cut the cod in 6-7 oz filets

Place the cut fish, sliced garlic, and sliced onions in a large bowl. Coat with 2 tbsp of olive oil, and a heavy pinch of salt, approx. 1/2 tsp. Toss to coat, and place on the side.

Line the pot or pan with 2 layers of parchment. Add in the crushed tomatoes and chicken broth.

Layer in the onions, garlic, and fish in the pan, making sure you are putting a good amount of the onions under the fish.
Add the tomatoes, and both olives, making sure they are for the most part resting in the sauce. Sprinkle the parsley and oregano and another 1/2 tsp of salt.
Place the pot on the stove on low-medium heat and cook for 17-23 minutes or until fish is cooked through and flakey. Serve over rice or with crusty bread.

VEGETABLE SALMON DELIGHT

PREP TIME: 10 minutes minutes
COOK TIME: 10 minutes minutes
SERVINGS: 2
CALORIES: 310 kcal

EQUIPMENT
Knife
Chopping board
wok or frying pan
Spatula
INGREDIENTS
100 g white cabbage
100 g tenderstem broccoli
1 large clove garlic
2.5 cm ginger
4 padrón chillies optional, shishito can also be used, or just bell peppers
½ Tbsp vegetable oil (or sesame or chilli oil)
2 salmon filets preferably skin on, so the fish stays intact
1 Tbsp light soy sauce
½ Tbsp oyster sauce
juice of half a lemon (or lime)
INSTRUCTIONS
Prep Work
Rinse then slice the white cabbage thinly.
Trim any unsightly ends off the broccoli and slice any that are particularly large.
Lie the garlic flat on your chopping board, and with the side of your knife, bash down hard on the garlic. Peel off

the skin and discard, we'll be using the garlic as it is, bruised and in 2-3 piece. Or one, if it remained whole, it doesn't matter.

Thinly slice the ginger.

Let's get Cooking

Heat the oil in a medium-large wok or frying pan, on medium heat.

Fry the garlic and ginger for 30 seconds.

Toss in the cabbage, tenderstem broccoli, chillies (if using), soy sauce and oyster sauce. Stir to mix well and bring up to a simmer.

Leave to cook, uncovered, over a low flame for 3 minutes. If your vegetables are getting dry, add a splash of water.

Increase the heat to medium-low, and push the vegetables to the side. Place the 2 salmon filets, skin side up, in the middle. Leave to cook for 2 minutes.

Very gently, turn the salmon over, so skin side down, and cook for another 3 – 5 minutes. This will depend on the thickness of your fish as well as how well done you like it. I like to finish mine when the middle is still a touch pink.

Pile some of the vegetable over the salmon to add a little flavor.

When done, take it off the heat and finish with the lemon juice drizzled over, and freshly ground black pepper and serve as discussed in the post (with any grain or on its own, as a low carb meal).

You could also finish it with a light drizzle of sesame oil or chili oil.

CREAMY SHRIMP PASTA

PREP TIME: 10 minutes
COOK TIME: 15 minutes
TOTAL TIME: 25 minutes

INGREDIENTS

3/4 lb fettuccine pasta
1 lb large raw shrimp, peeled and deveined (21-25 ct)
1 Tbsp olive oil
1/2 onion, (medium), finely chopped
2 Tbsp unsalted butter
1 garlic clove, minced
1/3 cup white wine, I used Chardonnay
2 cups whipping cream
1/3 cup shredded parmesan cheese
1/2 tsp Sea salt, or to taste
1/4 tsp black pepper, or to taste
1/4 tsp paprika, or to taste
1 Tbsp Parsley, finely chopped, to garnish

INSTRUCTIONS

Add 3/4 lb pasta to a pot of boiling water with 1 Tbsp salt and cook according to package instructions until al-dente. Drain without rinsing and set aside.

While pasta is cooking, prepare the shrimp and sauce. Season shrimp with 1/2 tsp salt, 1/4 tsp black pepper and 1/4 tsp paprika. Place a large, non-stick pan over medium/high heat and add 1 Tbsp oil. Once oil is hot, add shrimp in a single layer and cook 2 min per side or just until cooked through and no longer translucent. Remove to a separate dish to prevent overcooking.

In the same hot pan, add 2 Tbsp butter with finely chopped onion and sauté until soft and golden (3-5 mins), stirring often. Add minced garlic and sauté another minute until fragrant. Stir in 1/3 cup white wine and boil down until there is only 25% of the liquid left.

Stir in 2 cups cream, bring to a light boil then simmer 2 min. Sprinkle sauce with 1/3 cup parmesan cheese and stir just until creamy and smooth. Let it come just to a simmer without boiling then turn off the heat and season sauce with more salt, pepper and paprika to taste.

Stir in the drained pasta and cooked shrimp, tossing until noodles are well coated in sauce. Serve in warm pasta bowls with a generous sprinkle of finely chopped parsley, more parmesan cheese and some freshly cracked black pepper.

NOTES

Important: do not boil the alfredo sauce once the cheese is in, or the cheese will separate from the cream.

ROSEMARY BUTTERY FISH MEAL

SERVINGS: 2 servings
PREP TIME: 5minutes
COOKING TIME: 15minutes
TOTAL TIME: 20minutes

INGREDIENTS
Whitefish filet: 400 gms
Rosemary: 2 sprigs rosemary
Butter: 1 tbsp
Olive oil: 1 tbsp
Salt to taste
Crushed pepper: 1 tbsp
Lemon: juice of 1 medium-size lemon
Gluten-Free white flour for dusting (Optional)

INSTRUCTION
Wash the fish filets.
Dust the fish with a thin layer of gluten-free flour. This will make the skin a little crispy when you cook the fish in oil.
Now in a pan, heat some olive oil. Place the fish filets in (do not put all the pieces together, divide them into 2 batches), press the fish gently into the pan with a flat spatula, and cook over high (but not raging) heat until the underside turns golden brown one side.
Now add the salt, crushed pepper and cook on low-medium heat. When the underside turns dark brown, flip the fish over.

After you have flipped the fish, wait for the fish to turn light brown, now add the butter and one rosemary sprig to the pan. When the butter melts, spoon the butter over the fish with a spoon so that the butter covers the fish evenly and all over.

Cook the fish on medium-low heat for some time. When you see the underside is well cooked, take the fish off the heat. Squeeze some lemon on the cooked fish, serve with baked or grilled veggies.

CHAPTER 9 : BEYOND THE COOKBOOK

Maintaining your weight loss Success

Congratulations on your success in losing weight! Presently, imagine yourself as a talented director, coordinating an orchestra of sound decisions. The Weight Watchers cookbook turns into your printed music, directing you through an agreeable excursion.

First, treat the recipes as your diverse, flavorful, and balanced musical notes. Prepare healthy grains, lean proteins, and fresh produce with the right tools in your kitchen. Practice segment control; consider it keeping up with the right mood in your culinary execution.

Keep in touch with the people who help and inspire you, your support network. Like any gifted artist, practice consistency. Ordinary activity turns into the consistent beat, supporting your recently discovered wellbeing.

Keep in mind, periodic deviations resemble melodic extemporization they add suddenness to your excursion. Celebrate achievements; every accomplishment is a victorious crescendo in your weight reduction ensemble. You're not simply keeping up with weight; you're coordinating a way of life that sings with wellbeing and essentialness. Continue to lead, maestro!

Bouns : Exercise ideal
Flexibility and mobility exercises
Practice these:

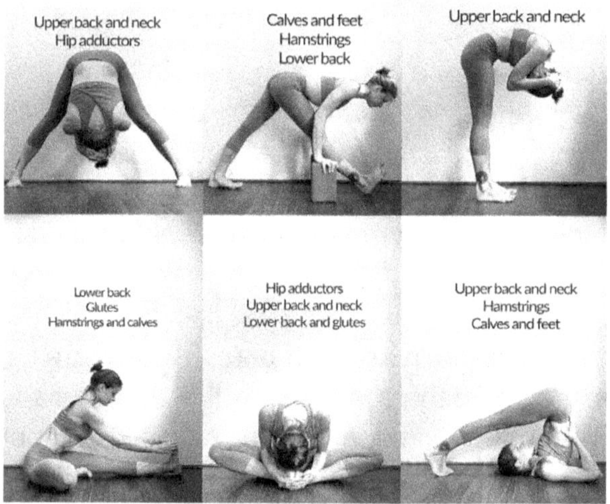

Let's delve into the dynamic duo of flexibility and mobility exercises a powerful synergy that not only enhances your weight loss journey but transforms the way your body moves and feels. Join me as we unravel the intricacies of when and how to incorporate these exercises into your daily routine for optimal results.

Firstly, let's talk timing. I've discovered that the beauty of flexibility and mobility exercises lies in their adaptability to various moments of your day. Consider incorporating them into your warm-up routine before a workout. This primes your muscles and joints, making your exercise regimen more effective while reducing the risk of injury.

Post-workout is another ideal window. I've felt the immediate relief of stretching after a workout, aiding muscle recovery and promoting flexibility gains.

But don't limit these exercises to just workout sessions I've found that incorporating short bursts of flexibility and mobility exercises throughout the day works wonders. Whether it's a quick stretch break at your desk or a few mobility movements before bed, these snippets add up, enhancing overall flexibility and fostering a sense of well-being.

Now, let's explore the 'how.' Flexibility exercises, like static stretches, are fantastic for elongating muscles and increasing range of motion. I've weaved them into my routine, focusing on major muscle groups such as hamstrings, quadriceps, and shoulders. Hold each stretch for about 15-30 seconds, breathing deeply to encourage relaxation.

On the flip side, mobility exercises involve dynamic movements that engage joints through their full range of motion. Think leg swings, arm circles, or hip rotations I've found joy in these fluid motions that not only improve mobility but also elevate heart rate, contributing to calorie burn.

The secret sauce lies in consistency. I've realized that the effectiveness of flexibility and mobility exercises is tied to making them a consistent part of your routine. Aim for at least 10-15 minutes a day, gradually increasing duration and intensity as your flexibility improves.

As you embark on your weight loss journey, view flexibility and mobility exercises not as additional tasks but as essential components. I've experienced firsthand the positive impact they have on weight loss by enhancing overall movement efficiency and making physical activity more enjoyable.

Incorporate these exercises thoughtfully, listen to your body, and relish in the newfound agility and freedom they bring to your weight loss journey. Here's to a flexible, mobile, and vibrant you.

Core and stability exercises

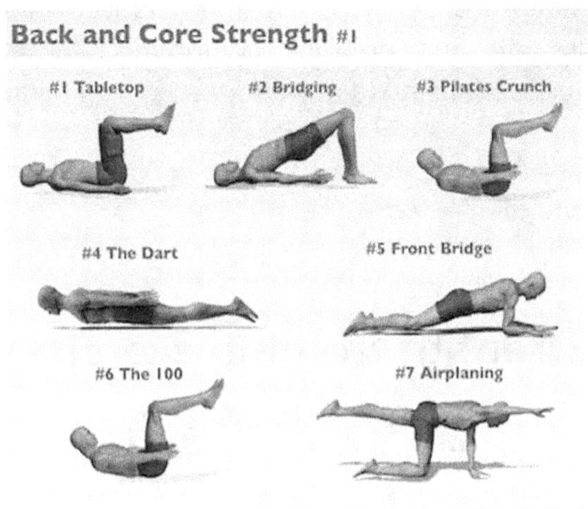

Core exercises focus on strengthening the muscles in your torso, including your abdomen, back, and pelvis. These muscles play a crucial role in supporting your spine, maintaining proper posture, and facilitating everyday movements. Stability exercises, often integrated with core workouts, enhance your body's ability to control and stabilize various movements.

When performing core exercises, it's essential to engage your abdominal muscles and maintain proper form to maximize effectiveness. Common exercises include planks, crunches, and leg raises. Stability exercises may involve balance challenges, using tools like stability balls or balance boards.

Incorporate these exercises into your routine 2-3 times a week. Start with foundational moves, gradually progressing in difficulty. Consistency is key for building core strength and stability, contributing to improved overall functional fitness and reduced risk of injuries.

Strength training exercises

STRENGTH TRAINING
Workout Routine

Do 3 sets of 12 reps in each round resting 30 seconds in between.

Round 1:
Squat to Overhead Press
Chest Flies
Tricep Kickbacks

Round 2:
Curtsy Lunge to Leg Lift
Bicep Curls
Deadlifts

Round 3:
Kettlebell Squats
Kettlebell Upright Rows
Kettlebell Bent Rows

Strength training involves lifting weights or using resistance to build and tone muscles. When you lift weights, your muscles experience microscopic damage. As your body repairs these microtears, it adds more muscle fibers, leading to increased strength and size over time.

To get started with strength training, establish a routine that targets major muscle groups, including legs, chest, back, arms, and core. Use a mix of compound exercises (working multiple muscle groups) and isolation exercises (focusing on specific muscles).

Begin with a warm-up to increase blood flow and flexibility. Gradually increase the weight as your strength improves, aiming for 2-3 sets of 8-12 repetitions per exercise. Allow your muscles at least 48 hours of rest between sessions.

Focus on proper form to prevent injuries, and consider working with a fitness professional or trainer to ensure a well-rounded and safe program. Consistency is crucial, so aim for 2-3 strength training sessions per week to see noticeable results in strength, muscle tone, and overall fitness

CARDIOVASCULAR EXERCISE

Benefits of Cardiovascular Exercise

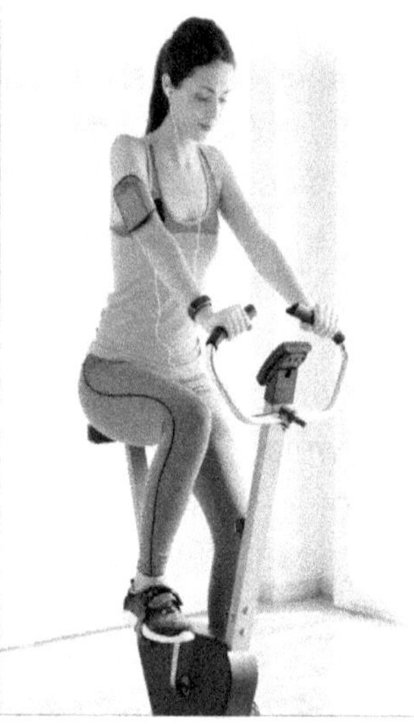

Improved Blood Circulation: Improved blood flow aids in the delivery of oxygen and nutrients to cells as well as the removal of waste materials.

Weight Management: Cardio workouts burn calories, which aids in weight loss and management.

HEALTHY FACTS

Imagine your body as a finely-tuned instrument, and cardiovascular exercise as the rhythm that keeps it in harmony. Start by choosing activities you enjoy, turning the beat into a dance rather than a chore. Begin with a warm-up think of it as tuning your instrument before the main performance.

Consider mornings as the overture a refreshing start to your day with activities like jogging or brisk walking. It's like setting the tempo for the day ahead. If evenings are more your style, treat it as a closing act, releasing the day's stress through activities like cycling or swimming.

Consistency is your melody; aim for at least 150 minutes per week, turning cardiovascular exercise into a regular part of your life's soundtrack. Listen to your body's tempo increase the intensity gradually, like elevating the volume in a crescendo.

it's not just about burning calories; it's about pumping vitality into your cardiovascular system. Find your rhythm, and let the symphony of a healthy heart play on!

CONCLUSION

In the tempting universe of the "New Weight Watcher Cookbook," every recipe is a delicious section in your own health story. This culinary journey elevates the routine into the extraordinary with vibrant salads, hearty main courses, and guilt-free desserts.

You will discover that this cookbook is not just about losing weight; rather, it is a road map to a lifestyle in which nourishing your body is a delightful adventure rather than a chore as you explore the tantalizing flavors and smart, mindful choices.

Therefore, let these recipes serve as your compass, leading you toward a life that is both balanced and full of life. Whether you're a carefully prepared gourmet specialist or a kitchen fledgling, leave on this culinary journey with energy and relish the compensating taste of a better, more joyful you. Not only is the "New Weight Watcher Cookbook" a book, but it's your buddy in making an account of wellbeing, each flavorful dish in turn.

ABOUT THE AUTHOR

Dr. Sharon S. Lent

Welcome to the realm of sustainable weight loss and nourishing diets! Dr. Lent, a seasoned medical professional specializing in weight loss and diet, brings a wealth of expertise to guide you on your transformative journey to a healthier you.

Meet Dr. Sharon S. Lent

With a passion for empowering individuals to achieve their health goals, Dr. Sharon S. Lent has dedicated her career to the intersection of medicine, nutrition, and well-being. Holding a Doctor of Medicine degree, her specialized focus on weight loss has allowed her to make a meaningful impact on countless lives.

Areas of Expertise

Dr. Lent is renowned for her comprehensive approach to weight management, combining medical knowledge with practical, sustainable strategies. Her expertise includes personalized diet plans, evidence-based interventions, and holistic well-being practices.

A Trusted Guide:

As a trusted guide on the journey to better health, Dr. Lent emphasizes the importance of mindful living, making choices that resonate with individual lifestyles, and fostering a positive relationship with food.

Contributions to the Field:

Beyond her clinical practice, Dr. Lent is an avid contributor to the field of weight management. Her research, articles, and contributions to reputable health publications reflect a commitment to sharing knowledge and fostering a community dedicated to wellness.

Join the Journey:
Embark on a journey towards sustainable weight loss and a nourished, balanced life with Dr. Lent. Through her insights, you'll discover practical, achievable steps that go beyond the conventional approach to dieting, paving the way for a healthier, more vibrant future.

REVIEW

Dear **Reader,**

We hope you're enjoying your journey with the "Keto Smart diet 2024" Your experience matters to us, and we'd love to hear your thoughts on how the program has been for you.

Whether you've just started or are well into your transformation, your review can inspire others and help us fine-tune our approach to better suit your needs. Please take a moment to share your feedback on the "Keto Smart diet 2024". Your insights are invaluable in shaping the success stories of our community.

Thank you for being a part of this journey with us. Your review is not just a reflection of your experience but also a beacon for others seeking a healthier lifestyle.

We appreciate your time and input.